Negative Calorie Diet & Anti-Inflammatory Diet Guide

LELA GIBSON

LELA GIBSON

CONTENTS

LELA GIBSON

LELA GIBSON

Negative Calorie Diet

Cookbook & Guide Which Will Help You To Burn Body Fat, Lose Weight And Live Healthy

Lela Gibson

LELA GIBSON

Introduction

I would like to thank you for buying the book, *"Negative Calorie Diet"*.

This book contains proven steps and strategies on how to burn body fat, lose weight and eat healthy.

Are you on the verge of giving up on your weight loss goals? Have you tried reducing your fat intake, eating fewer carbohydrates and all the diets that call for eating fewer proteins and carbohydrates, drank a lot of water, but you don't lose any weight? Does nothing seem to work?Well, I guess losing hope is understandable, but wait, DO NOT GIVE UP JUST YET! There is one more option, the best option in fact: *The Negative Calorie Diet.*

If we are to go by the facts, theNegative Calorie Diet is the fastest way to lose weight; you can lose up to 14 pounds a week when you adopt the diet! Thanks to this diet, losing weight is no longer a random dream or a hope; it is a reality for thousands of people across the globe.

In this book, you will learn more about the Negative Calorie Diet, how it works and some amazing recipes that will help you burn fat.

Thanks again for buying this book, I hope you enjoy it!

Negative Calorie Diet: What Is It

This unique diet draws upon theidea that some foodshave the 'negative calorie' effect that we ought to consider in burning fat. A food is considered to have a negative calorie effect when the calories these foods use to digest are typically higherthan the calories in the foods themselves.

When you eat something, you begin by chewing, a process that consumes energy. Some foods such as those higher in stringy fibers like celery will require more chewing, which will result in more energy expenditure, and there are otherslike pasta and cakes that don't require as much chewing.

After chewing, the foods go to the stomach through the esophagus and the other processes of digestion take over until absorption takes place and the body excretes the residual mass.

With negative calorie foods, this entire process uses up more calories than the foods have. The extra calories the body has to provide in order to process the foods are taken from the fat stores, and the more of these negative calorie foods you eat, the more your fat stores will lose calories, and as a result, the more fatyou will lose.

Let us take broccoli as an example: 100 grams (contains 25 calories).

When you eat 100 grams of broccoli, it takes your body about 80 calories worth of energy to digest it. This results in a net calorie use of 55 calories that should come from the fat stores in your body. As you can see, the 55 calories make up the negative net calorie.

Let us now take a counter example of a piece of cake containing 400 calories.

Your body will take about 150 calories to digest the piece of cake, leaving net 250 caloriesdeposited in the body and stored as fat.

The negative calorie diet consists of over 100 foods proven to have negative calorie qualities. Most of these foods are fruits and veggies that are high in fiber. Let us look at them in more detail in the following chapter.

Negative Calorie Food List

Here is a list of negative calorie foods:

Vegetables

Vegetables are highly nutritious and not high in calories when compared to many processed foods. Nonetheless, some vegetables are superior especially when it comes to the negative calorie food list. The following are vegetables you should consider including in your diet.

Artichokes	Bean sprouts	Broccoli	Cabbage	Cauliflower
Asparagus	Beets and beet greens	Brussels sprouts	Carrots	Celery
Chives	Cucumbers	Green beans	Mushrooms	Peppers (red, green, yellow)
Pumpkin	Sauerkraut	Spinach	String beans	Turnips
Corn	Eggplant	Lettuce	Peas	Pickles
Radishes	Scallions	Squash	Tomatoes	Zucchini
Garlic	Onion	Watercress		

Fruits

Just like vegetables, fruits are a healthier option and always the recommended healthy alternative to sugary foods. It is therefore a better idea to snack on a bunch of grapes than it is to snack on candy.

However, when it comes to fruit choices, you also need to make better choices because some fruits are high in calories; thus, not providing you the negative calorie effect you are looking for in negative calorie foods

The list below contains some good negative-calorie fruits you can eat:

Apples	Blackberries	Cantaloupe	Cranberries	Grapefruit
Honeydew melon	Lemons	Mangoes	Apricots	Blueberries
Cherries	Currants	Grapes	Kiwi	Limes
Nectarines	Oranges	Pears	Pomegranates	Strawberries
Watermelon	Peaches	Pineapple	Raspberries	Tangerines
Prunes				

Herbs and Spices

When it is a question of what you eat, even herbs and spices matter. Below is a complete list of herbs and spices you should always go for.

Chili pepper	Cloves	Ginger	Parsley	Cinnamon
Mustard seeds	Cayenne	Anise	Coriander/ Cilantro	Dill
Cumin	Fennel seeds			

Meat, Fish and Seafood

Red meat can be harmful to you, and many negative calorie diets don't recommend it; however, you do not have to avoid eating meat altogether, as it provides essential proteins and other nutrients. A good source of protein is fish for instance. Fish is lower in calories but high in essential nutrients like omega-3 fatty acids.

If you are allergic to fish, or if you are not a big fan of it, you can alternatively include small/reasonable potions of meat and chicken in your diet (I will teach you how in the recipes section).

The table below shows some of the best fish and seafood to include in your diet:

Clams	Crayfish	Mussels	Shrimp	Crab
Flounder	Tuna	Abalone	Buffalo fish	Cod
Terrapin	Bass	Catfish	Trout	

How To Make The Transition To Negative Calorie Diet

Now that you know what to eat, let us see exactly how you are going to be eating all that.

1. Make a smooth transition into the negative calorie diet so that you are comfortable with the entire process. Start by adding some negative calorie foods to the foods you normally eat in every meal in the 1:1 ratio. For instance, if having pasta with meatballs, you can serve 50% of this food and add chunks of zucchini to fill the other half.

You can also add a mixed salad to each meal you have; the salad should comprise of not less than 90% negative calorie foods. This means you have to look for ways to substitute any unwanted content such as any creamy high-fat substances with something like raspberry vinaigrette.

After some time, start slowly substituting the foods with the good (negative calorie) ones until your plate contains up to 90% negative calorie foods.

Note: We are only adding vegetables and fruits so far, not necessarily fully prepared negative calorie meals. Next, we will discuss the recipes so that you have entirely cooked meals too.

2.Use several vegetables to make a stir-fry. You can also make smoothie shakes with your favorite fruits including some berries. As said before, the negative calorie diet is largely a fruits and vegetables diet. However, this does not mean you should now start worrying about how you will survive as a vegetarian.

You can occasionallyenjoy small servings of chicken and some meat, and the recipes in the following chapter will reflect that. Nonetheless, the meats have to be in small amounts; remember, you are losing weight and so, you have to make some sacrifices.

First Thing to Do

Buy all the foods you think you require from the list, wash, cut them into bits then seal them in airtight containers for storage (in the fridge) so that you will have them handy anytime you need them. You do not want to come home from work tired in the evening without having a bunch of these foods readily available. If you do, you will be extremely tempted to grab something unhealthy.

If you are wondering whether you will be hungry on this diet plan, just know that you will not because these foods are filling because they are high in fiber as well as water; the perfect combination to be full.

Second Thing To Do

One thing you will discover as you start the negative calorie diet is that it is not easy to give up eating some foods. This is especially so if you've formed bad eating habits through the years. Habits such as eating in front of the television and snacking on junk food may be difficult to break. However, you have to do it.

This brings us to the second thing you need to do.

You need to get rid of foods that do not adhere to the negative calorie diet. As they say, out of sight, out of mind. Once you determine which foods to eat, the next thing is removing the foods that are not part of the diet. However, this does not mean that you need to get rid of such foods all at once.

Second Thing To Do

One thing you will discover as you start the negative calorie diet is that it is not easy to give up eating some foods. This is especially so if you've formed bad eating habits through the years. Habits such as eating in front of the television and snacking on junk food may be difficult to break. However, you have to do it.

This brings us to the second thing you need to do.

You need to get rid of foods that do not adhere to the negative calorie diet. As they say, out of sight, out of mind. Once you determine which foods to eat, the next thing is removing the foods that are not part of the diet. However, this does not mean that you need to get rid of such foods all at once.

As has been said, you should gradually shift to the negative calorie diet. You can't do this if you get rid of every food you should not eat. This means that you must determine how to go about doing away with such foods. Start by listing the foods down and then go about eliminating a few of the foods from your diet each week. This way, you will soon find yourself eating only the foods approved by the negative calorie diet.

Note: While on this diet, you should have no room for alcohol, sugar, or any sugar substitutes except stevia simply because sugar intake causes your body to produce more insulin. This hormone signals/tells the fat cells to pick up and convert any excess glucose into fat. Therefore, eating more sugar means more production of insulin and consequently, more deposits in the fat cells. We are trying to reduce fat in your body, not create more of it. In this regard, avoid all commercial dressings since most of them contain sugar and high fat content.

Third Thing To Do

The next step is to plan your meals. If you think about it, you usually have an idea of what you want to eat for breakfast, lunch and dinner. Unfortunately, you may have to stop eating many of those foods. This means you need to figure out what you will eat during meal times. This is where meal planning comes in.

Meal planning involves looking at your diet and determining which foods will go well together. When you are on the negative calorie diet, you find yourself enjoying a variety of fruits and vegetables. This is a nice opportunity to make different types of salads. Salads are easy to make and they contain many valuable nutrients. However, you can easily get bored if you eat the same type of salad day in, day out. This is why it makes sense to take a moment to plan your meals.

Meal planning is also quite useful when it comes to doing your shopping. As we have said, fruits and vegetables will feature prominently in your diet. You will want to use fresh produce as much as possible. This means you should time your shopping properly. If you determine which meals you'll be preparing beforehand, you can go ahead and shop for particular foods instead of shopping without a plan. This will ensure you have what you need when you need it.

Now that we have that out of the way, let us start cooking!

Negative Calorie Diet Recipes

While on a strict diet (such as this one), you might have a problem trying to decide what kind of dressing to use for your meals. Since I know it is important to be careful about what you are using, I will start by giving you two simple dressings that you will use on any meal you want.

Garlic and Herbs Dressing

Mix 1/2 cup of cold-pressed extra-virgin olive oil with juice from 1 lemon, 2 crushed garlic cloves and ¼ cup apple cider vinegar. Add some of your favorite negative caloriedried herbs such as parsley and cilantro.

This will yield 1 cup of dressing. Store the dressing in the fridge (for up to one month) to use on your foods.

Dijon and Yoghurt Dressing

For a delicious vegetable dip, mix Dijon mustard (2 tablespoons) with 2 cups low-fat yoghurt then add a pinch of chili pepper and a teaspoon of mixed dried herbs to spice it up.

Breakfast Recipes

Pumpkin Pancakes

Serves 4

Ingredients

1 cup of canned pumpkin

1 1/4 cups of water

2 teaspoons of cinnamon

2 cups Krusteaz pancake mix

1 egg, slightly beaten

1 teaspoon of baking powder

For the topping

1/4 cup of sliced pecans

5 tablespoons of pure maple syrup

Instructions

Combine all the ingredients for the pancake batter.

On a griddle or pan over medium heat sprayed with a little cooking spray, create a 10 cm circle of batter.

When the pancakes turn brown at the edges and you notice even bubbling across the top, flip them over to cook the other side.

In the meantime, toast pecans in a small pan until they turn slightly brown and give out the fragrance.

Serve with heated pure maple syrup.

Apple and Cinnamon with Almonds and Oat Bran

Serves 4

Ingredients

4 large apples

1 teaspoon of ground cinnamon

1/4 cup of oat bran

10 almonds, toasted and chopped

1 teaspoon of unrefined coconut oil

2 cups of unsweetened vanilla almond milk

2 packets monk fruit extract

Instructions

Wash the apples and cut into cubes.

Melt the coconut oil in a large nonstick skillet over medium high heat. Add the cinnamon and apples then cook for 2-3 minutes until the apples soften.

Remove from the heat, add almond milk, stir in the monk fruit extract and oat bran. Once mixed return back to the heat, stir, and bring to a simmer.

Cook for about one minute, until the mixture becomes thick and creamy.

Divide the mixture among four bowls then sprinkle each one with toasted almonds.

Negative Calorie Smoothie

Serves 2

Ingredients

5 strawberries

½ medium papaya

1 grapefruit

¼ cup ice

Instructions

Put all the ingredients in a blender; blend until smooth.

Serve and garnish with some strawberries and enjoy.

Lunch Recipes

Vegetable Soup

Serves 6

This is not your regular veggie soup; yes, it is simple, but it is full of negative calorie foods only.

Ingredients

6 cups of vegetable stock

1 cup of celery, diced

1 cup of green beans cut into about 1 inch pieces

1 medium zucchini, diced (approximately 2 cups)

1 cup small turnip, diced

1 jalapeno, seeded and finely chopped

1 medium onion, diced

1 cup of cauliflower florets

2 cups of shredded cabbage

3 cloves of garlic, finely chopped

2 cups of baby spinach

Salt and pepper to taste

Instructions

Mix the ingredients (except the spinach) in a pot, and bring to a boil.

Cover and let it simmer for 20 minutes.

Add the spinach, stir, and let it cook for one more minute.

Remove from the heat and serve.

Toast with Tomatoes

Serves 4

Ingredients

8 cups of spinach

½ ripe avocado, mashed well with a fork

Salt to taste

Freshly ground black pepper to taste

4 slices of natural gluten-free bread

4 (½-inch) slices ripe tomato

4 eggs, poached

Green hot sauce

Instructions

Place a nonstick skillet over medium high heat.

Add the spinach and cook until it wilts. Move the spinach to a colander and strain out as much water as possible. Put the now drained spinach in a bowl and season with green hot sauce and salt.

Use a toaster to toast the bread then season the avocado with salt. Evenly spreadthe pieces of avocado over each piece of toast then add a slice of tomato on top. Use pepper and salt to season the tomatoes and use the spinach mixture to top each slice evenly.

Place every piece of toast on a fresh plate. Finally, top with a poached egg and serve.

Meatballs with Mushroom Gravy

Serves 4

Ingredients

12 ounces lean ground beef

1 ounce Parmigiano Reggiano cheese, finely chopped

2 tablespoons arrowroot, dissolved in 2 teaspoons of stock

8 cups washed spinach

1 cup thinly sliced onion

4 cups sliced cremini mushrooms

Olive oil cooking spray

Freshly ground black pepper

Salt to taste

4 cups unsalted beef stock

1 cup finely chopped puffed brown rice

Instructions

Put the beef in a large bowl and push it to one side. Add rice and a cup of the stock to the other side of the mixing bowl; season with pepper and salt and allow the rice to absorb the stock for about 1 minute.

Mix the beef and rice using an electric hand mixture until well mixed. Taste and adjust the seasoning then use the mixture to form 16 meatballs.

Coat a skillet with olive oil cooking spray and place over medium heat. Once hot, put the meatballs and brown for one minute on one side. Turn and brown the opposite side for around 30 seconds and transfer to a plate.

Add the mushrooms to the skillet and sauté for a few minutes. Add the meatballs back to the skillet, then add the beef stock, arrowroot mixture, and cook until meatballs are cooked through.

Add the spinach and season with pepper and salt and cook until the spinach is wilted. Add the cheese, stir, and serve.

Dinner Recipes

Brussels Sprouts with Lemon and Almond Dressing

Serves 3-4

Ingredients

3 pints Brussels sprouts, shaved thinly

5 teaspoons of freshly minced garlic

Crushed red pepper flakes

1/2 cup of chopped fresh flat-leaf parsley

Salt

1 1/2 teaspoons of extra-virgin olive oil

1/4 cup of toasted almonds, finely chopped

1/8 teaspoon of ground cinnamon

1/2 cup freshly squeezed lemon juice

1 ounce of Parmigiano-Reggiano cheese, finely grated

Instructions

Place the Brussels in a large mixing bowl and place it aside.

Placea non-stick skillet over medium high heat then add the garlic and olive oil. Cook until the garlic turns deep golden brown. Remove from the heat then add the parsley, almonds, cinnamon, and red pepper flakes.

Return the skillet back to the heat sauté for about ten seconds.Remove from the heat, pour in the lemon juice, and then season with salt.

Add the dressing to the Brussels then toss well, add 75% of the cheese, and toss some more. Taste then add the seasoning and top with the rest of the cheese.

Chicken with Pesto

Serves 3 or 4

Ingredients

Water

6 garlic cloves, chopped

Dash of paprika

1 cup of fresh basil leaves

8 cups ofchopped escarole

Salt

1 ounce of Parmigiano-Reggiano cheese, finely grated

Olive oil cooking spray

Dash of cinnamon

Crushed red pepper flakes

1 small onion, thinly sliced

4 cups chicken stock,unsalted

12 ounces of skinless, boneless chicken breast sliced into 1/8 inch thick strips

Instructions

Pour 2 quarts of water in a medium pot and bring to a simmer. You will use this to poach the chicken.

Lightly coat a medium skillet with olive oil cooking spray then place it over medium high heat.

Add the garlic and cook until it turns golden brown. Add the cinnamon, basil leaves, red pepper flakes, onion, and paprika. Cook for roughly 2 minutes until the onion softens.

Add the escarole then cook until it is soft and wilted – for 2 more minutes. Add the stock, bring to a simmer, and then cover. Cook for about 5 minutes or until tender.

Add a pinch of salt to the simmering water and turn off the heat. Add the chicken and stir well until all parts separate. Cook until you notice the strips turning white (meaning they are half cooked). Use a slotted spoon to transfer the strips to a plate to cool.

Let the remaining mixture cook until most of the stock evaporates and looks like thick sauce or soup. Turn off the heat.

Add in half of the cheese, stir, and then season with salt to taste. Add the chicken strips then toss them to coat with the mixture and keep cooking until the strips have cooked enough through, for about 90 seconds.

Top with the remaining cheese, and then serve.

Vegetable Beef Soup

Serves 14

Note: This recipe has many ingredients and it is likely you will hate some vegetables or herbs. You can replace these vegetables and herbs with other ingredients on the negative calorie food list.

Ingredients

4 chopped onions

1 chopped red bell pepper

4 cups of sliced fresh mushrooms

10 chopped celery stalks with their leaves

2 cupsof fresh chopped broccoli

1 small chopped bunch of cilantro

5 box low sodium beef broth

1 large chopped green bell pepper

4 cups of chopped cabbage

6 large chopped fresh carrots

1 finely chopped head of garlic

6 cups of fresh chopped spinach

1 small bunch of Parsley

1 canof asparagus (drained)

2 cans of green beans (drained)

1 cupof canned artichokes (drained)

20 twists of cracked black pepper

1 tablespoon of Italian seasoning

Protein (you can use just about any meat preferably the fishes mentioned in the list)

2 10 oz. cans of tomatoes with green chili's (not drained)

2 cans of diced tomatoes with basil (not drained)

1/2 tablespoon of red pepper flakes

1 tablespoonof dried basil

2 small cans of chopped green chilies (not drained)

1 lb. 80/20 or leaner ground beef (drain if needed)

Instructions

Fill a large cooking pot halfway with the beef, chicken, or vegetable stock. Add all the canned ingredients while draining some as specified intothe pot.

Add water and all the spices then stir. Let it boil for some time, lower the heat to simmer for one hour or until the vegetables soften.

As the soup boils down, add some extra broth and stir.

Serve, garnish as desired, and enjoy.

Snacks

Apple Chips

Serves 2

Ingredients

2 large granny smith apples

1 teaspoon of stevia

1 teaspoon of cinnamon

Canola oil cooking spray

Instructions

Preheat your oven to 200 degrees.

Using a sharp knife, thinlyslice the apples crosswise. Arrange the slices on a single layer on a baking sheet then spray with canola oil cooking spray.

Evenlysprinkle the stevia and cinnamon over the apple slices.

Use the bottom third part of the oven to bake the apples until they are crisp and dry, roughly 2-2½ hours.

Alternatively, you could use a mastrad chipmaker. Not only is it easy and fast, you do not need the cooking spray. Just lay the apple slices on the chipmaker, sprinkle with cinnamon and stevia, and then microwave for 4-5 minutes.

Berry Salad

Serves 4

Ingredients

4 cups of mixed berries (blackberries, raspberries, blueberries, strawberries)

20 whole almonds, toasted and chopped

2 tablespoons of hemp hearts

1/4 cup of cooked quinoa

1 ½ tablespoons of fat free yoghurt

Instructions

Equally divide all the ingredients among four bowls and toss well to mix.

Fruit Salad

Serves 10

Ingredients

2/3 cup of fresh orange juice

1/2 teaspoon of grated lemon zest

2 cups of cubed fresh pineapple

3 kiwi fruits, peeled and sliced

2 oranges, peeled and sectioned

2 cups of blueberries

1/3 cup of fresh lemon juice

1/2 teaspoon of grated orange zest

1 teaspoon of vanilla extract

2 cups of strawberries, hulled and sliced

3 bananas, sliced

1 cup seedless grapes

Instructions

Add orange zest, orange juice, lemon juice and lemon zest, to a saucepan, place it over medium high heat, and bring to boil.

Decrease the heat to medium-low and let it simmer for 5 minutes. Remove from the heat and stir in the vanilla extract. Place it aside to cool.

Place the fruit in a clear glass bowl in layers starting with the pineapple, then strawberries, kiwi, bananas, oranges, then grapes and at the top, blueberries.

Pour the juice over the fruit layers then cover and leave in the fridge for 3-4 hours before serving.

Almond Cake with Berries

Serves 4

Ingredients

½ cup of almond meal

4 packets of monk fruit extract

1 teaspoon of vanilla extract

Olive oil cooking spray

2 eggs, separated; remove 1 yolk

3 tablespoons of raw coconut nectar

Salt

1 cup of mixed berries, mashed well with a fork

Instructions

Preheat your oven to 3750 degrees F.

Bake the almond meal until it becomes aromatic and well toasted —about 3-5 minutes. Remove from the oven and place it on a cool baking sheet.

Place the monk fruit and egg whites in a bowl and whisk until it forms stiff peaks. Use cooking spray to spray four paper cups. Using a toothpick or fork, poke holes in the bottom of each.

Place the almond meal into a mixing bowl then add the egg yolk, salt, vanilla, and coconut nectar. Fold the meringue into the mixture of almond and transfer the batter into the cups.

Place in the microwave and microwave for about thirty seconds. When the mixture has cooked through, place the cups on their sides and give them 45 seconds to cook.

Remove the cakes and place themupside down on four serving plates.

Get them off the cups and serve with berries.

Cucumber and salsa

Serves 2

Ingredients

2 cucumbers, peeled and sliced

12 garlic cloves, minced

¼ cup fresh cilantro, chopped

3 tomatoes, diced

½ sweet onion, diced

Sea salt and black pepper to taste

Instructions

Mix all ingredients except the cucumber in a bowl in order to make the salsa.

Place cucumber slices on a plate and serve with the salsa.

Negative Calorie Diet And Exercise: An Effective Way To Lose Weight Fast

I promised you some unique and cool exercise tips, right? Doing the following exercises will help you burn the fat much faster. All you have to do is to start slow and over time, increase the intensity, keep an open mind, and use the gym (for the ones that require it), where you have an instructor nearby.

Interval Training

This is all about high intensity exercises combined with short periods of rest. This will not only burn more calories than your typical cardio training, it will boost your body's ability to burn fat easily since it increases the production of the growth hormone, which is also a fat burning hormone, and adrenaline which assists in suppressing your appetite.

The intervals will work on your muscles, and help them use oxygen better so that your heart does not have to struggle to pump a lot to make them perform.

Do It!

Get on a treadmill or a stationary bike then use the guide below to start your own interval-training regimen:

Begin with a regular warm-up (any simple exercise to get your blood rushing). When done, run or pedal at a rate that is more than your regular cardio intensity by 20%. If you have never engaged in any serious cardio workouts before, you might want to check this first to understand what I am talking about.

After 30 seconds to 1 minute, reduce the intensity to a rate that is 50% less than the intensity of a regular cardio workout. Alternate the periods of 30 seconds to 1 minute of hard work with 30 seconds to 1 minute of relaxed pedaling or if you want, relaxed running for 6-10 intervals to finish your session.

As this gets simpler, increase each interval's intensity so that you work even longer during the difficult part, reduce your rest periods, or if you feel enthusiastic enough, add more intervals.

Repeat 3-4 times each week.

As you get the hang of this exercise, start the next:

Sprinting

Try sprinting up a hill since the impact on your joints will be much lower and can help you avoid injury. If there is no hilly ground in your area, try the alternative: the dag race approach. Start your sprint by increasing your speed from a jog.

To make the most of this exercise, keep the sprints short – ideally50 yards per sprint. This helps you sustain a high intensity all through and prevents injury.

If you want to increase the overall results of your sprint workout, increase your total number of sprints. This is better than going for long distance runs.

If you are new to exercising, do not do more than one workout per week. You can increase the days once you accustom to the exercise; just remember to allow at least two days of recovery between the workouts.

As you get the hang of the above exercise, start the next:

High Intensity Strength Intervals

Select two exercises that work different muscles completely or ones that use opposite movements. For instance, you can pair a pulling exercise with a pushing exercise or upper body exercise with a lower body exercise like pull-ups and squats.

For the latter, select a weight (if your instructor thinks you need one) with which you can do 10 repetitions. Alternate between the two exercises and do just five repetitions of each move in every set. Remember to rest between the sets so that you finish each set without failing.

Keep alternating between the exercises for a 10 or 15 minutes set time. Keep noting the total number of sets you can do. In subsequent sessions, try to beat your score by completing more sets in the same duration or completing the same number of sets but with heavier weights.

As you get the hang of the above exercises, start the next:

Countdown Workouts

Countdown workouts fit in the use of exercise pairs really well. They also keep you fully engaged in the exercises since you have to keep the count and pay attention.

With every round of the exercise pair, the training encompasses one lesser rep of each move; for instance, you move from a set of six to five…until zero.

You can also try density training where you pair opposing exercises for countdowns. For instance, kettlebell swing, pushups, and squat thrusts would work really well.

Do it!

Start by selecting your pair of exercises.

Perform six repetitions of the first exercise, then six reps of the other move. Go back to the first move and perform five reps then five more of the second exercise. Keep alternating until you reach zero.

In the subsequent workouts, add one rep to each exercise. If you want more countdowns, select a second pair from the list below, or just come up with your own pair of opposing moves.

Squat thrust, pushups

Kettlebell swing, squat thrust

Jumping jacks, pushups

Medicine ball side toss, medicine ball slam

As you get the hang of the above exercise, start the next:

Hurricane Workouts

This is essentially a workout protocol that entails lifting weights and interval training. We have three groups of exercises, called rounds in this type of workouts. Each round has an exercise that increases your heart rate, and a set of other exercises in between.

This design will allow you to keep your heart rate up throughout the workout (and burn significant amounts of calories) that typically lasts 16-22 minutes. Hurricane workouts have five levels and each one is an increased challenge. I have however prepared for you a sample routine you will work with below.

Note: This will require you to be more fit- if fit enough though, you can begin with this:

Warm up for the workout. For all rounds, do one set of each exercise and move on to the next exercise. Finish the whole round thrice before you move to the next round.

First round: Run on a treadmill at 10% incline, 10.5 mph for 25 seconds. Do a kettlebell Turkish getup about 4 times on each side of your body then 10 chin-ups.

Repeat this sequence thrice.

Second round: Run on a treadmill at a 10% incline, 11 mph for 25 seconds. Do 10 dips and a barbell rollout, 15 reps.

Repeat this process thrice.

Third round: Run on a treadmill at a 10% incline, 11.5 mph for 25 seconds. Perform the G.I row, 10 reps. Do the knee grab, 20 reps.

Repeat three times.

I need your help...

Thank you for buying this book!

I hope this book was able to help you to know more about the Negative Calorie Diet and how you can burn fat and lose weight with this diet, the next step is to put what you have learned into practice and actually adopt the diet if you want to see those pounds coming off.

Finally, if you enjoyed this book, then I'd like to ask you for a favor, would you be kind enough to leave a review for this book on Amazon? It'd be greatly appreciated!

I want to reach as many people as I can with this book, and more reviews will help me accomplish that!

If you have any questions or problems, please contact us: hello@freedomdestination.com

Thank you and good luck!

Anti-Inflammatory Diet Guide

The Guide To Reduce Inflammation And Live A Healthy Life Without Pain

LELA GIBSON

LELA GIBSON

INTRODUCTION

I want to thank you and congratulate you for buying the book, *"Anti-Inflammatory Diet Guide"*.

This book contains proven steps and strategies on how to reduce inflammation and live a healthy life without pain.

Each day, we expose our bodies to chemicals, processed foods high in additives and other unhealthy ingredients as well as other pollutants. It is no wonder that suffering from inflammation is quite common.

For most people, the first thing they do once they discover that they are suffering from inflammation is to reach for drugs. However, the thing about drugs is that they address the symptoms associated with inflammation. Therefore, if you want to deal with the problem, you need to address the root cause of inflammation. One of the main causes of inflammation is our diet.

In this book, you will learn more about inflammation and the anti-inflammatory diet that you need to embrace if you want to treat inflammation.

Thanks again for buying this book, I hope you enjoy it!

CONTENTS

Effects Of Inflammation

Inflammation is the biological response your body goes into when dealing with harmful stimuli such as irritants, pathogens or even damaged cells. It is a self-protection mechanism that allows your body to begin the healing process. The 'hotness' or 'inflammation' you feel after you cut yourself or injure yourself is the result of your body working hard to heal itself. But what happens when your body experiences 'too much' inflammation?

A little inflammation is not a bad thing. In fact, when it happens, you should rejoice in knowing that your body is working tirelessly to correct the situation. However, like most good things, inflammation can get out of hand. When this happens, you may experience various health complications such as:

Weight Gain

Every day, thousands of people try to lose weight to no avail. They complain that they've tried out various diets but somehow none seem to be working. If they do find something that works, sooner than later, they are back to gaining the weight they thought they'd lost. This is because they neglect to look into inflammation as the cause for their weight gain. Inflammation contributes to weight gain in various ways. These include:

- If inflammation happens in the brain, it interferes with the functioning of the hypothalamus and this in turn increases your appetite and slows down your metabolism. When this happens, you will be eating a lot but burning up less energy, which leads to weight gain.

- Gut inflammation leads to leptin and insulin resistance. Leptin is the satiety hormone that tells your brain when you have had enough. When suffering from leptin resistance, you just eat and eat some more before leptin can communicate that you have had enough, which leads to weight gain. Another thing that gut inflammation does is to increase intestinal permeability. When this happens, more toxins will be able to permeate your bloodstream. Usually toxins are stored in fat cells to remove them from circulation. The more toxins you have, the more the fat cells expand to accommodate the more toxins leading to weight gain.

- Inflammation in the endocrine system suppresses adrenal and thyroid function. One of the main functions of the adrenal gland is to burn fat. Therefore, when you suppress the functioning of the adrenal gland, you are unable to burn fat, as you should leading to weight gain.

As you have read, inflammation is bad for you if you want to maintain the ideal weight.

Metabolic Syndrome

Metabolic syndrome refers to a group/cluster of lifestyle-related diseases including cardiovascular disease and obesity. They are clustered together because all of these diseases are linked to metabolic dysfunction. Markers of metabolic dysfunction include:

- Central obesity – this is excessive tummy fat

- Hyperinsulinaemia – this refers to ongoing high levels of insulin

- Insulin resistance –your body loses sensitivity to insulin (you need more insulin to manage your blood sugar levels)

But the question is how these three factors are connected. Well, when on a diet high in carbohydrates, your blood sugar levels increase leading to high insulin levels to help blood cells absorb the glucose and thus manage your blood sugar levels. When you have high insulin levels, the production of cytokines (which are pro-inflammatory) increases and in turn this causes inflammation especially in predisposed persons. Once inflammation increases, it brings with it an increase in the production of free radicals. Free radicals affect cellular functions and one of those functions just happens to be insulin sensitivity. This is why chroni low-grade inflammation is linked to all three markers; that is, raised insulin levels, obesity and decreased insulin sensitivity.

Chronic Fatigue

Many people suffering from chronic fatigue have been told that the disease 'is all in their minds'. Fortunately, in recent years more researchers have began looking into the association of chronic fatigue and inflammation. This is mainly because the two possess many similar symptoms including muscular pain and tenderness, sore throat, joint pain, swollen lymph nodes and sore throat.

As you know, inflammation is the way your body reacts to foreign particles. When you have symptoms of inflammation, it is safe to say that your body is fighting something even if that something is not yet known. This is why researchers link an overactive immune system to chronic fatigue.

Another thing that associates chronic fatigue with inflammation is the lack of cortisol in patients suffering from chronic fatigue. Cortisol is known to suppress inflammation. Thus, if your body has a cortisol deficiency, it will not be able to suppress inflammation and this will worsen symptoms of chronic fatigue. A dietary change often helps people suffering from chronic fatigue.

Some types of arthritis

When you hear the name arthritis, you automatically associate it with pain. Well, it is no coincidence since arthritis refers to inflammation in joints. When your joints experience inflammation, you will feel pain. The types of arthritis that have been linked to inflammation include:

- Gouty arthritis

- Rheumatoid arthritis

- Psoriatic arthritis

- Systematic lupus erythematosus

When you suffer from these types of arthritis, you may experience inflammation symptoms such as redness, joint stiffness, swelling of the joints, pain in the joints and loss of joint function.

It is important to note that inflammation does not have to be painful for it to be present. This is because many organs in your body just don't have enough pain-sensitive areas for you to feel that inflammatory sensation. This means that you can suffer from chronic inflammation over time without knowing, only for you to experience the effects of inflammation.

It is also important to note that various things can cause inflammation including:

- Processed foods high in sugar and unhealthy fats

- Omega-6 fats (and not enough Omega-3 fatty acids)

- Sleep deprivation

- Chronic stress

- Smoking

- Pollution

- Environmental chemicals

- Lack of exercise

Thus, chances are, if you experience any of the above things, you may be suffering from inflammation whether or not you experience pain.

The first thing you should do once you notice that you suffer from inflammation is not to reach for drugs because drugs just address the symptoms and not the root cause but rather to make some lifestyle changes. This is because most of the causes of inflammation can be addressed by making lifestyle changes like exercising more, reducing exposure to pollutants, not smoking and dietary changes.

In this book, we will focus on addressing inflammation by adopting an anti-inflammatory diet. Let us learn more about anti-inflammatory diet in the next chapter.

Anti-Inflammatory Diet: The Solution To Inflammation

An anti-inflammatory diet is a diet that is designed to reduce inflammation. Unlike most diets, it is not a one-size-fits-all diet. But it does include the dos and don'ts to guide you on how to proceed.

This means, it is up to you to check out the 'dos' or foods that have anti-inflammatory properties so that you can customize the diet according to your needs. For example, the diet recommends eating whole grains including wheat. However, some people don't react well to gluten. This means, they may not include gluten in their diet. However, they can certainly include other foods on the allowed foods list.

Other foods that have anti-inflammatory properties include fruits, vegetables, beans and foods that contain Omega-3s. You should also avoid foods that have inflammatory properties like highly processed foods, foods high in sugar and unhealthy fats.

It is important to point out that the anti-inflammatory diet is not a diet per say but rather a lifestyle change. You will be making a conscious decision to reduce the sources of inflammation. Let us learn more about how an anti-inflammatory diet will help address inflammation.

How An Anti-Inflammatory Diet Suppresses Inflammation

It is important to understand how the anti-inflammatory diet works in order to be motivated to adopt the diet. Several related things affect inflammation. These are:

Free radicals

As you know, the human body is composed of cells. In turn, these cells are composed of molecules. The molecules consist of atoms. These atoms have elements joined by chemical bonds. The strength of the bonds determines the stability of the molecules.

Weak bonds often split leading to 'free radicals' that can quickly react with other compounds in order to gain stability. In the course of doing this, the free radicals can displace other molecules, 'stealing' their electrons and this can lead to a chain reaction that can cause disastrous effects by disrupting a living cell.

It is important to note that while free radicals are formed normally during metabolism, certain factors such as eating certain foods, daily stress, processed foods, smoking, pollution, drugs, some herbicides and radiation can also lead to the spawning of free radicals. When the free radicals become too many, it leads to oxidative stress.

Oxidative stress

Your body is built in such a way that it neutralizes and processes free radicals. Unfortunately, when the free radicals are too many, your body will be unable to neutralize them. It will become overwhelmed and this will create an imbalance. This imbalance is what it referred to as oxidative stress and it leads to inflammation.

Inflammation

Many experts suspect that oxidative stress is responsible for starting a bio-chemical cascade that leads to inflammation and other degenerative diseases. Remember I mentioned earlier that free radicals could overwhelm the system.

Think of your body like a computer. You can use it to perform many tasks. When you open one or two programs or documents, you have no trouble performing the tasks that will lead to getting the outcome you desire. However, what happens when you open 10 or more programs to deal with various tasks? Suddenly your computer becomes too slow. It becomes overheated.

The same can happen to your body if it has too many radicals. It becomes inflamed. When this happens, you will need antioxidants to bring down the inflammation. This is where the anti-inflammatory diet comes in.

Antioxidants

Antioxidants, which can be found in various antioxidant rich foods, work well to trap or neutralize free radicals. Antioxidants 'donate' their electrons such that free radicals are forced to bond to them. This stops the electron stealing reaction. It also protects cells from the damage caused by free radicals 'stealing' their electrons.

When free radicals are too many, they wreak havoc in your body. They cause damage and lead to oxidative stress, which leads to inflammation. Thus, neutralizing free radicals is the key to reducing inflammation. An anti-inflammatory diet contains many foods that are rich in antioxidants that can effectively reduce inflammation.

In summary, an anti-inflammatory diet does away with foods that cause oxidative stress while encouraging you to eat foods rich in antioxidants. When you follow this diet, you will effectively neutralize free radicals, prevent oxidative stress and consequently reduce inflammation. This is why it is important to know what to eat and what not to eat.

Anti-Inflammatory Diet: What To Eat

As we've seen, various things can trigger inflammation. There is no reason you should add on to this by eating foods that cause inflammation. In fact, by eating anti-inflammatory foods you can help your body deal with inflammation. Below are some anti-inflammatory foods that you should include in your diet

Fruits and Vegetables

Fruits and vegetables are rich in anti-inflammatory antioxidants and should feature prominently in your diet. Below are some of the best fruits and vegetables for treating inflammation:

Dark, leafy greens

Dark, leafy greens such as kale, romaine and spinach are great for reducing inflammation because they are rich in antioxidants. Kale contains quercetin and Kaempferol antioxidants while romaine contains carotenoids and spinach contains the antioxidant lutein. They are also equipped with other anti-inflammatory agents. You can enjoy such vegetables in salads and smoothies.

Blueberries

Fruits have anti-inflammatory vitamins, Vitamin A, Vitamin C and Vitamin E. These are great at helping your body repair itself. Blueberries also contain the powerful antioxidant anthocyanin, which is great for fighting inflammation. Eat the berries as a snack or add them to your salad and smoothies.

Cruciferous veggies

Cruciferous veggies such as broccoli, cabbage, kale and cauliflower are loaded with antioxidants such as lutein, zeaxanthin and carotenoids. This means they can successfully reduce inflammation and the symptoms associated with it. Make it a habit to increase your consumption of such vegetables. You can even include them in juices and smoothies.

Avocados

Avocados are great for reducing inflammation because they are high in carotenoids. Carotenoids fight inflammation. However, as always, you need to be careful when consuming avocados. Don't overdo it. Half a medium avocado per day should be enough for you. Anymore and you'll start adding on the pounds. You can eat it, as it is, add it to your salad or make guacamole if you'd like.

Asparagus

Asparagus is said to be a super anti-inflammatory food. This is because it has various anti-inflammatory nutrients such as asparanin A, quercetin, diosgenin, rutin, protodioscin, isorhamnetin, kaempferol and sarsasapogenin. Asparagus also has antioxidants. This makes it very useful in the fight against inflammation.

Beetroot

Beetroot is another important food you should include in your diet. It has anti-inflammatory benefits along other properties. Beetroot has phytonutrients such as isobetanin, betanin and vulgaxanthin that are linked to heart health. As you know by now, heart disease is also categorized as a symptom of chronic inflammation. You can include beetroot in salads and juices.

Herbs and Spices
Ginger

Ginger is a well-known spice among chefs. Apart from adding flavour to foods and tea, it is used for its healing properties. It contains anti-oxidants which are also good at fighting inflammation. You can sprinkle a dash of ginger onto your tea and soups whenever you like. This will increase your consumption of this useful spice.

Garlic

Garlic has been linked to various health benefits such as cardiovascular health and prevention of obesity and arthritis. It also has anti-inflammatory properties. Garlic contains the compounds thiacremonone and vinyldithin, which are good at inhibiting inflammatory messenger molecules. Allicin, a compound in garlic, also has many anti-inflammatory benefits. You can use garlic in various foods, salads and soups.

Turmeric

Turmeric is a chef's best friend because it not only adds flavour to food but it also adds colour. Another thing it is known for is its anti-inflammatory properties. You can put it in your vegetables and soup. But take note that turmeric is a bit pungent. If you're not used to it, start with using a little at a time and gradually increase the content.

Whole grains

Fiber is known to help fight inflammation. Whole grains are high in fiber. Eat foods high in fiber such as brown rice, oatmeal and whole-wheat bread. However, you should be careful to ensure that your body does not react negatively to the gluten contained in wheat.

Beans and nuts

Beans are also high in fiber and they have antioxidants. They also contain other anti-inflammatory properties that will prove quite useful to you. Nuts are also good for reducing inflammation. They are high in healthy fats that work to stop inflammation. A handful of nuts per day should be enough for you.

Foods Rich in Omega 3

Omega 3 fatty acids are great in fighting inflammation. Flaxseed contains this fatty acid and is especially good for the cardiovascular system. It also serves as a building block for molecules that work to prevent inflammation. Apart from that, omega 3 has been shown to prevent inflammation-based diseases such as depression, inflammatory bowel syndrome, diabetes, heart disease, asthma, osteoporosis and rheumatoid arthritis.

Apart from eating flaxseed, you should also eat fish and seafood. Endeavour to eat at least two servings each week.Herring sardines and salmon should feature in your diet as well as walnuts.

Chia seeds are also high in omega-3 fatty acids. You can add chia seeds to your salads and soups.

Supplements

You can also take supplements to reduce inflammation. These include:

- Spirulina – these algae is known for its strong antioxidant effects. It works to reduce inflammation and strengthen the immune system. You just need to take 1-8 grams per day.

- Resveratrol – this antioxidant can be found in fruits with purple skin such as blueberries and grapes. It is used to reduce inflammation in people who suffer from gastritis, heart disease, ulcerative colitis and insulin resistance. Take 150-500mg in a day.

- Ginger – ginger can also be taken in supplement form. You only need to take 1-2 grams in a day.

- Curcumin – this is found in turmeric and is great at reducing inflammation. You can take up to 100-500mg of this supplement per day.

- Fish oil – you can take fish oil especially if you don't eat fish regularly. Fish oil contains the beneficial omega-3 fatty acids which decrease inflammation. Take 1-1.5 grams of fish oil supplements per day.

Before taking any supplements, you need to read the instructions carefully to ensure the supplements do not interfere with any medicines you are already taking.

Good Fat

You should be careful about the fats you consume. Stick to coconut oil, hemp seeds, avocados, extra-virgin oil, organic canola oil and oily cold water fish such as trout, tuna, salmon and mackerel.

Fiber Rich Food

Foods high in fiber are also great at reducing inflammation. You can eat foods such as barley, quinoa, okra, brown rice, lima beans, black beans, almonds, eggplant, lentils, acorn squash, figs, chia seeds and berries.

Remember that not everyone reacts to food in the same way. You should be careful to note how your body reacts to certain food. In addition, don't make any drastic changes, as this will prevent you from knowing which food is causing you problems. Also, remember that some foods may contain anti-inflammatory properties but they may also be high in fat. It would be best to consume such foods in moderation.

Anti-Inflammatory Diet: What Not To Eat

When you're trying to reduce inflammation, you will achieve greater by knowing which foods to stay away from. Some foods are pro-inflammatory and frankly, most of them are just not good for your general health. Some of these foods include:

Sugar

Taking sugar increases your blood sugar levels and as we have learned, high insulin levels can trigger inflammation. In addition, sugar encourages your body to release cytokines. These are inflammatory messengers that lead to inflammation. Avoid sugar, soda and other sweet drinks.

Red meat

When you eat red meat, a chemical called NEu5gc is produced. When this happens, your body goes into an inflammatory immune response to deal with the chemical. Therefore, you would do well to avoid this. You should also try to avoid processed red meat such as hot dogs. These are usually high in saturated fat, which often causes inflammation especially when you eat too much red meat.

Dairy

Many people add milk to their breakfast cereal each morning. We also love having some cookies with a glass of milk. However, if you want to treat inflammation, you need to reduce your intake of milk. Why, you may ask. This is because milk has allergens such as casein, which spark inflammation.

Additionally, about 60% of the world's population are unable to digest milk in the first place. How many times do parents accuse their kids of eating 'too much' ice cream when they complain of having stomach cramps and feeling gassy. Guess what? It could just be that the kids are lactose intolerant.

Taking dairy products can lead to inflammatory responses such as hives, breathing difficulties, stomach distress, diarrhoea, constipation, acne, and skin rashes. These are clearly symptoms you can do away with by staying away from dairy products.

Trans-fats and excessive Omega 6 fatty acids

The ratio of omega 3 to omega 6 in your diet should be 1:1 or there about. Unfortunately, many people do not consume enough omega 3 fatty acids in their diet but take too much omega 6s for instance by using polyunsaturated fats such as sunflower, corn oil, soybean oil and safflower. It is said that many people consume omega 3s and omega 6s in the ration 1:20. This brings about an imbalance that leads to, cellular damage, inflammation and pain.

Similarly, many people consume trans fat. Hydrogenated and partially hydrogenated fats should have no business in your diet as they contribute largely to inflammation.

Refined Carbohydrates

Refined carbohydrates are grouped among the 'high glycemic index foods'. These are foods that lead to rapid increases in blood sugar (hyperglycemia). Hyperglycemia is often linked with inflammatory diseases. It triggers the release of cytokines which are inflammatory molecules.

On the other hand, when you eat carbohydrates that have natural fiber and fat, you will experience fewer pro-inflammatory agents. Stick to such carbohydrates instead of consuming refined carbohydrates.

Foods that cause allergies

Just because a certain food is known to work well in treating inflammation does not mean that it will work well for you. Some foods cause allergic reactions and initiate an inflammatory response. For example, some people are intolerant to dairy and wheat (gluten). Such people would do well to stay away from such foods. This is why it is wise to add one or two things to your diet at a time. This way, you can gauge your body's reaction to the foods you are including in your diet.

Knowing what to eat and what not to eat is just part of the journey towards reducing inflammation. The next step is actually using that knowledge to make the needed changes and achieve success.

Strategies To Put You On The Path To Success

It is one thing to know that you should add more fruits and vegetables in your daily diet but it is another thing to actually do it. This is especially so if you are used to eating high-carb foods and getting take-out. Fortunately, there are strategies you can use to improve your diet.

Figure out ways to sneak in anti-inflammatory foods

One way to increase your intake of anti-inflammatory foods is to incorporate them into your existing meals. This way, you will make your meals healthier without feeling as if you are making many changes at the same time. You can:

- Add foods such as celery, turmeric, and beetroot to your juice.

- Add garlic and turmeric to sauces.

- Add gibgerm flax oil, chia seeds and turmeric to your smoothies. You can also add avocado.

- Add quinoa to soups for added fiber and asparagus, beetroot, celery, cauliflower, ginger and turmeric to make soups more anti-inflammatory.

- If you're making a salad, take the opportunity to add various veggies and fruits. You can also add anti-inflammatory herbs such as ginger. Use oils such as flax oil for your dressing.

Make a transition plan

Quitting 'cold turkey' is quite difficult. In fact, many who do so soon find themselves back to their old habits because they cannot handle the changes. Instead of trying to get rid of everything at once, you can work out a transition plan that will get you to where you want to be. To do so:

- List down all the foods you eat and that you should give up. Once you list down such foods, determine which two foods you will give up each month. Then proceed to cut back on those two foods until you completely eliminate them from your diet. For example, if you want to reduce your intake of dairy, you can reduce your intake to 5 times a week, then three times, then once and finally you can remove dairy from your diet.

- List down all the foods you should eat and begin to add them to your diet. Remember you will be cutting down on foods you should not eat. When you do this, you can substitute the foods you shouldn't eat with those that you should eat. For example, after giving up refined carbs, you can start including whole grains in your diet. This way, your meals won't change but their quality will.

- Start drinking more water and eating healthier snacks. Also, you should start watching your portions to ensure you not only eat the needed foods but that you also eat enough of them to make a substantial change.

The idea is to make lifelong changes that will allow you to leave a healthy life without pain. You can do this by making small and deliberate changes and pretty soon you will have developed good eating habits to last a lifetime.

Develop good eating habits

Eating habits are formed over time and they become so ingrained that you rarely think about them in detail. For example, you may find yourself always having coffee with toast for breakfast. It becomes your usual routine. Well, if you wish to be successful at reducing inflammation, you have to develop good eating habits that will allow you to do just that. One thing you can do is follow the anti-inflammatory diet pyramid developed by Dr. Joe Feuerstein (Columbia University). The pyramid indicates the foods you should eat starting from the bottom to the top level.

- Bottom level – Vegetables and fruits should feature prominently in your daily diet. Eat 2-3 fruits and 6-8 servings of veggies and salads every day.

- Level II - Whole grains and healthy carbs such as yams, plantains, whole grain pasta and quinoa should be eaten in limited amounts.

- Level III - Nuts and seeds should feature in your diet as should avocado, hemp and olive oils.

- Level IV - Proteins such as tofu, whole soy, tempeh, sardines, salmon, herring and sockeye should be eaten in moderation.

- Level V - This level includes foods such as eggs, bison, natural cheese and skinless poultry. These foods should be eaten in small amounts. Also, remember to remove the skin from any poultry you eat.

- Top level - The top level of the pyramid includes foods that you should eat in small amounts. These include things like dark chocolate and red wine.

When you change your eating habits to include various anti-inflammatory foods, you will start seeing the difference as you become healthier and pain-free. Forming a habit is a process. But it can be done and many have done it successfully, so can you. In addition, you can do other things to reduce inflammation.

Lower your calorie intake

Another thing that can help you address inflammation is reducing the amount of calories you eat. Eating fewer calories ensures you do away with diseases and conditions such as obesity, heart disease, type II diabetes. All these diseases have been linked to causing inflammation. A great way to reduce your calorie intake is to increase your vegetable intake and lower your intake of carbohydrates especially refined carbohydrates. This is because vegetables are high in fiber but very low in calories, which ensures you feel full. Vegetables are also rich in antioxidants. Therefore, when you increase your vegetable and fruit intake, you are taking foods rich in antioxidants, which will help in fighting inflammation.

Start Exercising

It is true that when you engage in bouts of exercise, your body experiences increased inflammation; you will suddenly find your joints and muscles aching. However, it is also true, if you continue engaging in regular exercise, you will be in the 'best shape' you've ever been in. This is because regular exercise decreases inflammation. Thus, instead of aiming high, you first need to lower your standards so that your body can get accustomed to the pace at which you are putting it through. As they say, don't run before you learn how to walk. Start by taking walks, increasing the distance and reducing the time for the walks. This way, your body will gradually adjust and before you know it, you will become fit and you will experience all the benefits that come with exercising.

Have adequate sleep

When you don't have enough sleep, you soon find yourself complaining of various ailments. The same goes when you sleep 'too much', you wake up with aching joints and complain of backaches among other ailments. When your sleep is disturbed, you also experience a variety of symptoms that bother you throughout the day. This clearly shows that the amount and quality of your sleep is linked to inflammation. Actually, insomnia and sleep disturbances increase the risk factor of inflammation.

Make sure that you get at least 7-8hours of uninterrupted sleep. Try coming up with a sleep schedule that will allow you to get the needed sleep. Set a nighttime routine and stick to it as much as you can so that your brain can adjust to the routine and prepare for sleep.

Keep a food journal

Some people love keeping journals. Others don't. But if you're tired of pain and discomfort, you will benefit greatly by having a food journal. This journal should focus on what you eat and how it makes you feel. The purpose of keeping a food journal is to discover what foods trigger inflammation in you as an individual.

Yes, you need to stay away from certain foods. This does not mean that your body will respond well to all the foods in the recommended food list. Individual circumstances may come into play to make certain foods unsuitable for you. In addition, there are a variety of foods around the world. The anti-inflammatory food list is by no means exhausted. If you come across some food not listed, you may decide to try it out and note down how it makes you feel. This way, you can customize your diet and continue to enjoy a variety of foods.

Establish a support system

Another thing you can do to succeed on the diet is establish a support system. It's not easy going on a diet. You have to make changes. You have to buy into it and find reasons to keep doing it. If you don't have a support system, you may forget why you're on the diet in the first place.

The amazing thing is that you can get support from family members and friends. But, first, you need to explain to them what you're doing and why you're doing it. This way, they will be supportive. Even if they don't join you on the diet, they will look out for you because they know the importance of the diet.

You can also find support from online groups and forums. Look around and determine with forum you're comfortable with. When you read about other people's journeys, you are likely to be motivated to stick to the diet. You can also share your story to keep yourself motivated and to motivate others.

Also, don't neglect to find strength in your own motivation. Think about your life and how you want to live it. Write down the reasons why you're sticking to the diet and use these reasons as motivation. You can have post-it notes at strategic places to remind you of what you have to gain. Thus, any time you want to falter, you'll have various reasons to keep going.

Live your life

Life does not stop just because you are on a diet. Nor should you expect it to. The anti-inflammatory diet should not keep you from enjoying your life or participating in various activities. It should not stop you from eating out with friends or going to social events. You can work your way around such things.

For example, if you're going to a social gathering, you can eat at home before heading to the event. This way, when you're there, you can stick to eating a salad without feeling left out. This will enable you to still enjoy the company of your friends without compromising your diet.

It would also be wise to practice beforehand what you will say to others about your diet. Many people are curious about such things and will want to know more. The good thing is that once they understand the diet, they may be your greatest allies. This will make your life easier and you will be able to enjoy a healthy life without pain.

At the end of it all, what you are trying to do is change your lifestyle so that you can live a healthy life without pain. When you eat anti-inflammatory foods, drink a lot of water, exercise and sleep well, you are giving your body the best chance to fight inflammation. This in turn leads to a healthy pain free life.

I need your help...

Thank you again for buying this book!

As you have learned, an anti-inflammatory diet is meant to stop or reduce inflammation. It does this by including foods rich in antioxidants and fiber and other anti-inflammatory properties. Fruits, vegetables, whole grains, fish and seafood are some of the foods you can use to reduce inflammation. In addition, reducing inflammation will help you reduce pain associated with inflammation and you can live a healthy life free of pain.

Finally, if you enjoyed this book, then I'd like to ask you for a favor, would you be kind enough to leave a review for this book on Amazon? It'd be greatly appreciated!

I want to reach as many people as I can with this book, and more reviews will help me accomplish that!

If you have any questions or problems, please contact us: hello@freedomdestination.com

Thank you and good luck!

Preview Of '20 Easy And Fast Diet Tips For Losing Weight'

Before we start learning about the strategies you can use to lose weight, let's start by highlighting some of the benefits that will come as a result of shedding those extra pounds just to give you extra motivation to want to do something NOW.

Why You Need To Lose Weight

Healthy weight loss has over one hundred benefits; these include emotional and physical benefits. I will dedicate this section to discussing the health benefits that many people (and weight loss/health books) do not pay enough attention to.

1: You Avoid Pre-Diabetes or Type 2 Diabetes

Pre-diabetes/high blood glucose is a condition that develops when the blood sugar levels in your blood move past normal ranges but not enough to qualify as diabetes. When your body stops consistently producing insulin sufficient to meet your body's needs, or the amount produced does not work properly, type 2 diabetes is likely to develop. Being pre-diabetic places you at a very high risk of developing type 2 diabetes.

Being obese or overweight is a proven leading risk factor for type 2 diabetes because carrying excess weight typically makes it hard for cells to respond to insulin, and since the additional fat acts as an insulating layer, it makes it more difficult for the sugar to enter the cells, which results in more circulating blood sugar levels.

Nonetheless, if you are already a pre-diabetic, you can prevent the progression to diabetes by shedding some weight (to reduce the insulating layer on cells so that they respond more to insulin) and trying to maintain a healthy weight.

2: You Keep Your Heart Healthy

When it comes to heart disease, some of the key risk factors are high cholesterol and high blood pressure. Research shows that:

1. Excessive accumulation of body fat makes your body release particular chemicals that occur naturally into the bloodstream, which increases blood pressure, and

2. Being overweight makes the liver produce too much amounts of Low density Lipoprotein (LDL) also called cholesterol. LDL tends to be sticky and gathers in the walls of blood vessels, which causes the narrowing of arteries, a condition called atherosclerosis, which increases your risk of strokes and heart attack.

When you lose weight, your blood pressure often reduces and the liver naturally reduces the amount of LDL it produces.

Royal Adelaide Hospital conducted a research on cardiovascular improvements with respect to a special weight loss program. Their results showed a decrease of cholesterol by 12%, a 10% decrease of LDL, a 5% decrease in diastolic blood pressure, and an 8% decrease in systolic blood pressure.

Check out the rest of 20 Easy And Fast Diet Tips For Losing Weight on Amazon, go to:**http://amzn.to/2kGyXvc**

Check Out My Other Books

Below you'll find some of my other popular books that are popular on Amazon and Kindle as well.

Alternatively, you can visit my author page on Amazon to see other work done by me.

20 Easy And Fast Diet Tips For Losing Weight – An Easy-To-Follow Weight Loss Guide

Belly Diet: The Zero Belly Diet Step-By-Step Guide Which Will Help You To Lose Your Belly And Enjoy Your Flat Belly

Dash Diet: Cookbook For Weight Loss With Action Plan And Easy Recipes

Clean Eating: Cookbook And Guide To Restore Your Body's Natural Balance And Eat Healthy

Negative Calorie Diet: Cookbook & Guide Which Help You To Burn Body Fat, Lose Weight And Live Healthy

Smart Fat: Cookbook With Fat Meals Which Help You To Lose Weight, Get Healthy And Improve Brain Function

www.ingramcontent.com/pod-product-compliance
Lightning Source LLC
Chambersburg PA
CBHW070026260726
48658CB00002B/508